By the year 2025 it is predicted t[...] have high blood pressure accord[...] HomeCare blog. And according [...] Americans eat comes from packaged, processed, store-bought, and restaurant foods. Only a small amount about 5% comes from salt added during cooking or at the table.

Americans consume an average of more than 3,400 milligrams (mg) of sodium each day. The _2015-2020 Dietary Guidelines for Americans_ recommend consuming less than 2,300 mg of sodium each day as part of a healthy meal plan. Although the American Heart Association recommends under 1500mgs.

The top six sources of sodium as reported by the American Heart Association include: breads and rolls, pizza, sandwiches, cold cuts and cured meats, soup and burritos and tacos.

This log book is designed to help you monitor the amount of sodium you're consuming from snacks and meals. Instead of guessing, it will provide a way for you to record the amount of sodium you are consuming on a daily basis.

Thank you for purchasing this log book. I hope you find it beneficial.

Emma

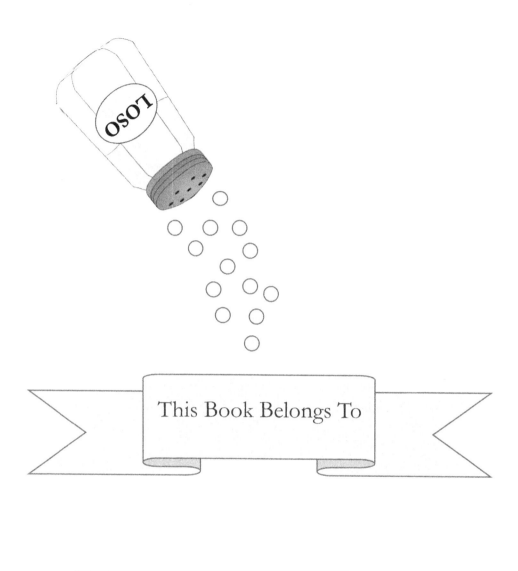

This Book Belongs To

What Is Your Sodium Level Goal? What Will It Mean To Me To Accomplish it?

_____

_____

_____

_____

_____

_____

_____

_____

_____

_____

_____

_____

_____

_____

_____

A Goal Without a Plan is Just a Wish

Date: 6/5/20

Mo__ Tu__ We__ Th__ Fr__ Sa✓ Su__

~~Breakfast~~

Food/ Beverage	Serving Size	Sodium	Calories	Protein	Carbs	Fat
2 eggs		140				
1 tsp		110				
1 tbs	mayo	100				
Coffee						
Yogurt			55			
Totals		350	405			

Snack

Serving size _____   _____ Protein

Sodium _____   _____ Carbs

Calories _____   _____ Fat

Notes

Misc. Info

dinner - Shrimp - 6   689
     pasta
      Summer squash

$$+ \ 405$$
$$1084$$
mg

Date: 6/6

Mo__ Tu__ We__ Th__ Fr__ Sa__ Su_✓

Lunch

Food/ Beverage	Serving Size	Sodium	Calories	Protein	Carbs	Fat
1 C cereal						
1/4 C milk						
fresh strawberries						
coffee						
yogurt			65			
Totals						

Snack

Serving size _____   _____ Protein

Sodium   _____   _____ Carbs

Calories   _____   _____ Fat

Notes

Misc. Info

pork chop	162
potato salad	117
tomato	6
asparagus	—
	279

Brownie

Date: 6/8

Mo ✓ Tu__ We__ Th__ Fr__ Sa__ Su__

Dinner

Food/ Beverage	Serving Size	Sodium	Calories	Protein	Carbs	Fat
Cereal						
blueberries						
milk						
square						
Totals						

yogurt

Snack

Serving size _____   _____ Protein

Sodium   _____   _____ Carbs

Calories   _____   _____ Fat

Notes

Misc. Info

dinner

steak
salad /dressing
pot salad
vegg

drink

Date: 6/9/20

Mo__ Tu✓ We__ Th__ Fr__ Sa__ Su__

Breakfast

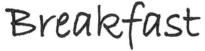

Food/ Beverage	Serving Size	Sodium	Calories	Protein	Carbs	Fat
1 C cereal		150				
1/4 C milk		25				
2 eggs	2x62	124				
1 tbs wheat tins		55				
Yogurt		75				
		429				
Totals						

Snack

Serving size _____   _____ Protein

Sodium   _____   _____ Carbs

Calories   _____   _____ Fat

Notes

Misc. Info

2000 mg

Dressing	280
Chit	85
Corn	—
Potato	117
Salad	
	482
Pie	195
Soda	5

Date: _____

Mo__ Tu__ We__ Th__ Fr__ Sa__ Su__

Lunch

Food/ Beverage	Serving Size	Sodium	Calories	Protein	Carbs	Fat
Totals						

Snack

Serving size _____   _____ Protein

Sodium   _____   _____ Carbs

Calories   _____   _____ Fat

Notes

Misc. Info — Natural Sodium OK

Fruits

Vegetables

Am Heart Assn. heart.org

dash diet

jarred - low sodium

Coral

Date: _____

Mo__ Tu__ We__ Th__ Fr__ Sa__ Su__

Dinner

Food/ Beverage	Serving Size	Sodium	Calories	Protein	Carbs	Fat
Cereal						
¼ C milk						
Strawberries						
Totals						

Snack

Serving size _____   _____ Protein

Sodium _____   _____ Carbs

Calories _____   _____ Fat

Notes

Choc McD   160

Misc. Info

Tuna panni

hot dog in Crescent roll
apple sauce
Salad

Date: _____

Mo__ Tu__ We__ Th__ Fr__ Sa__ Su__

Breakfast

Food/ Beverage	Serving Size	Sodium	Calories	Protein	Carbs	Fat
Cereal						
str	175					
milk						
Totals						

Snack

Serving size _____   _____ Protein

Sodium   _____   _____ Carbs

Calories   _____   _____ Fat

Notes

Misc. Info

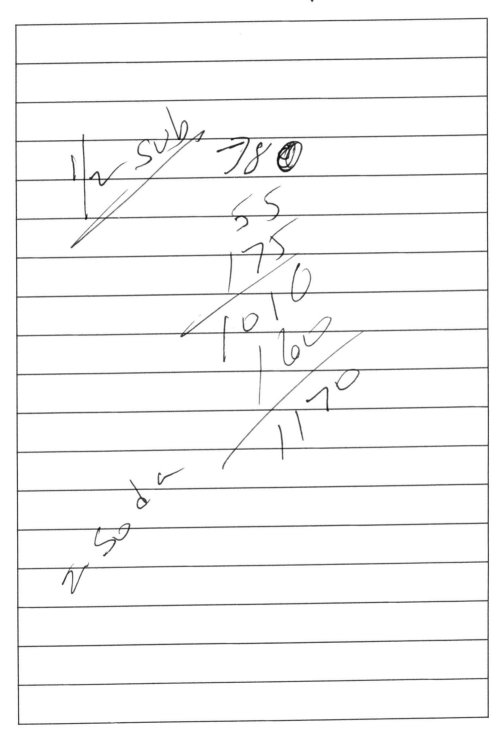

Date: ___6/12/20___

Mo__ Tu__ We__ Th__ Fr✓ Sa__ Su__

Lunch

Food/ Beverage	Serving Size	Sodium	Calories	Protein	Carbs	Fat
Totals						

Snack

Serving size _____   _____ Protein

Sodium   _____   _____ Carbs

Calories _____   _____ Fat

Notes

Misc. Info

780

Tuna Sand

Coffee

hot dog

apple sauce

salad

ranch dressing

Date: 6/13/20

Mo__ Tu__ We__ Th__ Fr__ Sa ✓ Su__

Dinner

Food/ Beverage	Serving Size	Sodium	Calories	Protein	Carbs	Fat
	Low fat					
1 Cup Cottch			660			
fruit						
			497			
burger						
Totals Salad						

eat Corn

Snack

Serving size _____

Sodium _____ 1 Tbs   2 mg

Calories _____

Protein

Carbs

Fat

Notes

tsp 2325

1/2 1162

Misc. Info

Date: ___6/14___

Mo__ Tu__ We__ Th__ Fr__ Sa__ Su__ ✓

Breakfast

Food/ Beverage	Serving Size	Sodium	Calories	Protein	Carbs	Fat
Totals						

Snack

Serving size _____   _____ Protein

Sodium _____   _____ Carbs

Calories _____   _____ Fat

Notes

Misc. Info

waffles	400
2 lbs butter 90 x 2	180
Syrup	210
	790

Coffee - med
    black (in)

slice pizza   1200

      1990 mg

Date: 6/15/20

Mo ✓ Tu__ We__ Th__ Fr__ Sa__ Su__

Lunch

Food/ Beverage	Serving Size	Sodium	Calories	Protein	Carbs	Fat
Totals						

Snack

Serving size _____   _____ Protein

Sodium _____   _____ Carbs

Calories _____   _____ Fat

Notes

Misc. Info

B/L

Cottage ch   660
peaches

Chili

12 Crakrs   100

Crispy sq   60
                 820

Date: __6/16/20__

Mo__ Tu_✓_We__ Th__ Fr__ Sa__ Su__

Dinner

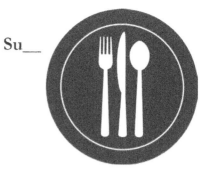

Food/ Beverage	Serving Size	Sodium	Calories	Protein	Carbs	Fat
Totals						

Snack

Serving size _____

Sodium _____

Calories _____

_____ Protein

_____ Carbs

_____ Fat

Notes

Misc. Info

banana

2 eggs / 2 slices bread

Date: _____

Mo__ Tu__ We__ Th__ Fr__ Sa__ Su__

Breakfast

Food/ Beverage	Serving Size	Sodium	Calories	Protein	Carbs	Fat
Totals						

Snack

Serving size _____

Sodium _____

Calories _____

_____ Protein

_____ Carbs

_____ Fat

Notes

Misc. Info

Banana

Crackers

2 HB eggs +
lettuce tomato

2 steak kabobs
Sauteed zucchini

Italian Ice

Date: __6|18__

Mo__ Tu__ We__ Th_✓_Fr__ Sa__ Su__

Lunch

Food/ Beverage	Serving Size	Sodium	Calories	Protein	Carbs	Fat
Totals						

Snack

Serving size _____   _____ Protein

Sodium _____   _____ Carbs

Calories _____   _____ Fat

Notes

Misc. Info

135
79

Ø 86

1 C low sod   110
    Cottage ch

fruit r lettuce)

2 burger
   ro ll   300
ketchup   180

soda

Date: _____

Mo__ Tu__ We__ Th__ Fr__ Sa__ Su__

Dinner

Food/ Beverage	Serving Size	Sodium	Calories	Protein	Carbs	Fat
Totals						

Snack

Serving size _____   _____ Protein

Sodium   _____   _____ Carbs

Calories   _____   _____ Fat

Notes

Misc. Info

291.6
126
/83

B'fast — black coffee
egg on english

Lunch   Salad
   greens, tom, feta ch
   greek dressing, 1 egg cuke

Snack

Dinner — roast chicken
   asparagus
   potato salad
   apple sauce

   jello + whip cream

Date: _____

Mo__ Tu__ We__ Th__ Fr__ Sa__ Su__

Breakfast

Food/ Beverage	Serving Size	Sodium	Calories	Protein	Carbs	Fat
Totals						

Snack

Serving size _____   _____ Protein

Sodium _____   _____ Carbs

Calories _____   _____ Fat

Notes

Misc. Info

291.8
112
78
82

B — cottage ch 1^C $\overset{2x}{55}$			110
Triscuit 6 = 50			100
Tomato 12			
juice 8g 140			210
12g 210			420

Cheddar bake   860
                     1280

Pork chops
mexican rice

Date: _____

Mo__ Tu__ We__ Th__ Fr__ Sa__ Su__

Lunch

Food/ Beverage	Serving Size	Sodium	Calories	Protein	Carbs	Fat
Totals						

Snack

Serving size _____   _____ Protein

Sodium   _____   _____ Carbs

Calories   _____   _____ Fat

Notes

Misc. Info

Waffle   400
butter - 2 tbs   180
Syrup 4 tbs =   7   Sod

potato salad
ratatouie
beef

Choc Cake

Date: __6/22__

Mo__ Tu__ We__ Th__ Fr__ Sa__ Su__

Dinner

Food/ Beverage	Serving Size	Sodium	Calories	Protein	Carbs	Fat
Totals						

Snack

Serving size _____

Sodium _____

Calories _____

_____ Protein

_____ Carbs

_____ Fat

Notes

Misc. Info

2   HB eggs
~~mayo~~
~~past~~
Coffee

lettuce ~~tom~~ cuke
egg
feta ch
dressing

did not eat all

pork
potato
mushroom

Date: **6/23**

Mo__ Tu_✓ We__ Th__ Fr__ Sa__ Su__

Breakfast

Food/ Beverage	Serving Size	Sodium	Calories	Protein	Carbs	Fat
Totals						

Snack

Serving size _____   _____ Protein

Sodium   _____   _____ Carbs

Calories   _____   _____ Fat

Notes

Misc. Info

2 eggs		140
2 toast	2 x 110	220
1 tbs mayo		100
		460

2 slice pizza	1200

spaghetti	167
home made marinara	1827

pt Janice
11:45-12

Date: ____6/24____

Mo__ Tu__ We✓ Th__ Fr__ Sa__ Su__

Lunch

Food/ Beverage	Serving Size	Sodium	Calories	Protein	Carbs	Fat
Totals						

Snack

Serving size _____   _____ Protein
Sodium _____   _____ Carbs
Calories _____   _____ Fat

Notes

Misc. Info

229.8

$\dfrac{150}{68}$ 84 ♡

3 pancakes →
butter
Syrup

Date: ___6/26___

Mo__ Tu__ We__ Th__ Fr✓ Sa__ Su__

Dinner

Food/ Beverage	Serving Size	Sodium	Calories	Protein	Carbs	Fat
Totals						

Snack

Serving size _____   _____ Protein

Sodium   _____   _____ Carbs

Calories _____   _____ Fat

Notes

Misc. Info 291.2

mayo	100
2 eggs	140
1 toast	110
Coffee	350
Salad —	
Crab cake	200
Lettuce, tom, cuke	
2 lbs ranch	260
Crispy square	60
	520

Date: 6/27

Mo__ Tu__ We__ Th__ Fr__ Sa✓ Su__

Breakfast

Food/ Beverage	Serving Size	Sodium	Calories	Protein	Carbs	Fat
Totals						

Snack

Serving size _____   _____ Protein
Sodium   _____   _____ Carbs
Calories   _____   _____ Fat

Notes

Misc. Info 290.2

Cereal, banana, milk

Date: __6/29__

Mo__ Tu__ We__ Th__ Fr__ Sa__ Su__

Lunch

Food/ Beverage	Serving Size	Sodium	Calories	Protein	Carbs	Fat
Totals						

Snack

Serving size _____   _____ Protein

Sodium _____   _____ Carbs

Calories _____   _____ Fat

Notes

Misc. Info

Anejo - margarita
tacos - guac
Swordfish   DQ

Strawberry Salad
(w chicken
Rasp Vin dressing   Zoo

Peach Pie

Date: __6/30__

Mo__ Tu_✓_We__ Th__ Fr__ Sa__ Su__

Dinner

Food/ Beverage	Serving Size	Sodium	Calories	Protein	Carbs	Fat
Totals						

Snack

Serving size _____   _____ Protein

Sodium   _____   _____ Carbs

Calories _____   _____ Fat

Notes

Misc. Info 292.°

B'fast coffee
½ tuna sand

Pot salad
Chix   dressing —
lettuc tom

green beans
meat loaf — squirt ketchup
pie

Date: _____

Mo__ Tu__ We__ Th__ Fr__ Sa__ Su__

Breakfast

Food/ Beverage	Serving Size	Sodium	Calories	Protein	Carbs	Fat
Totals						

Snack

Serving size _____   _____ Protein

Sodium   _____   _____ Carbs

Calories _____   _____ Fat

Notes

Misc. Info Sodium

pot salad

Yogurt   65

wings

Date: __7/2__

Mo__ Tu__ We__ Th√ Fr__ Sa__ Su__

Lunch

Food/ Beverage	Serving Size	Sodium	Calories	Protein	Carbs	Fat
Totals						

Snack

Serving size _____   _____ Protein

Sodium   _____   _____ Carbs

Calories   _____   _____ Fat

Notes

Misc. Info

Julie

293.2

B'fast

$\frac{118}{68}$

Cereal + milk

1/2 tuna sand
1 1/2 Slices bread
Lettuce Ham

Yogurt   50

hamburger
roll
mayo
tomato

apple sauce

Watermelon

Date: _7/3_

Mo__ Tu__ We__ Th__ Fr_✓_ Sa__ Su__

Dinner

Food/ Beverage	Serving Size	Sodium	Calories	Protein	Carbs	Fat
Totals						

Snack

Serving size _____   _____ Protein

Sodium _____   _____ Carbs

Calories _____   _____ Fat

Notes

Misc. Info   293
2000 mg

tuna sand   780
1 1/2 slices bread
lettuce tom

Yogurt   65

pork chop
potato - 1 tbs butter
broccoli

Watermelon

Date: __7/4__

Mo__ Tu__ We__ Th__ Fr__ Sa_✓_ Su__

Breakfast

Food/ Beverage	Serving Size	Sodium	Calories	Protein	Carbs	Fat
Totals						

Snack

Serving size _____   _____ Protein

Sodium   _____   _____ Carbs

Calories   _____   _____ Fat

Notes

Misc. Info

2000

2 pieces french toast	
(egg + milk)	220
maple syrup	7

Cabbage

rice

beef spare ribs

Date: __7/5__

Mo__ Tu__ We__ Th__ Fr__ Sa__ Su ✓

Lunch

Food/ Beverage	Serving Size	Sodium	Calories	Protein	Carbs	Fat
Totals						

Snack

Serving size _____   _____ Protein

Sodium   _____   _____ Carbs

Calories   _____   _____ Fat

Notes

Misc. Info

No B'fast

lunch —
    fr pineapple
     cottag ch   500
     lettuce
   Crackers - 16   55

Date: 7/18/20

Mo__ Tu__ We__ Th__ Fr__ Sa__ Su__

Dinner

Food/ Beverage	Serving Size	Sodium	Calories	Protein	Carbs	Fat
Crackers	8 oo	100				
Inst B.fst + milk	8 oz	220				
Totals						

Snack

Serving size _____   _____ Protein
Sodium   _____   _____ Carbs
Calories   _____   _____ Fat

Water 16 oz   Notes / in AM

Misc. Info

Date: 7/22

Mo__ Tu__ We✓ Th__ Fr__ Sa__ Su__

Breakfast

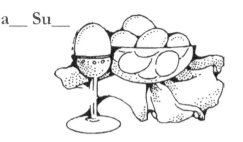

Food/ Beverage	Serving Size	Sodium	Calories	Protein	Carbs	Fat
Totals						

Snack

Serving size _____   _____ Protein
Sodium   _____   _____ Carbs
Calories   _____   _____ Fat

Notes

Misc. Info 290
2000 mg

Cereal + skim milk 200

Cottage 1/2 C
+ fruit   460   mg

Date: _____

Mo__ Tu__ We__ Th__ Fr__ Sa__ Su__

Lunch

Food/ Beverage	Serving Size	Sodium	Calories	Protein	Carbs	Fat
Totals						

Snack

Serving size _____   _____ Protein

Sodium _____   _____ Carbs

Calories _____   _____ Fat

Notes

Misc. Info

Date: _____

Mo__ Tu__ We__ Th__ Fr__ Sa__ Su__

Dinner

Food/ Beverage	Serving Size	Sodium	Calories	Protein	Carbs	Fat
Totals						

Snack

Serving size _____

Sodium _____

Calories _____

_____ Protein

_____ Carbs

_____ Fat

Notes

Misc. Info

Date: _____

Mo__ Tu__ We__ Th__ Fr__ Sa__ Su__

Breakfast

Food/ Beverage	Serving Size	Sodium	Calories	Protein	Carbs	Fat
Totals						

Snack

Serving size _____   _____ Protein

Sodium _____   _____ Carbs

Calories _____   _____ Fat

Notes

Misc. Info

Date: _____

Mo__ Tu__ We__ Th__ Fr__ Sa__ Su__

Lunch

Food/ Beverage	Serving Size	Sodium	Calories	Protein	Carbs	Fat
Totals						

Snack

Serving size _____   _____ Protein

Sodium   _____   _____ Carbs

Calories   _____   _____ Fat

Notes

Misc. Info

Date: _____

Mo__ Tu__ We__ Th__ Fr__ Sa__ Su__

Dinner

Food/ Beverage	Serving Size	Sodium	Calories	Protein	Carbs	Fat
Totals						

Snack

Serving size _____   _____ Protein

Sodium   _____   _____ Carbs

Calories   _____   _____ Fat

Notes

Misc. Info

Date: _____

Mo__ Tu__ We__ Th__ Fr__ Sa__ Su__

Breakfast

Food/ Beverage	Serving Size	Sodium	Calories	Protein	Carbs	Fat
Totals						

Snack

Serving size _____   _____ Protein

Sodium   _____   _____ Carbs

Calories   _____   _____ Fat

Notes

Misc. Info

Date: _____

Mo__ Tu__ We__ Th__ Fr__ Sa__ Su__

Lunch

Food/ Beverage	Serving Size	Sodium	Calories	Protein	Carbs	Fat
Totals						

Snack

Serving size _____

Sodium _____

Calories _____

_____ Protein

_____ Carbs

_____ Fat

Notes

Misc. Info

Date: _____

Mo__ Tu__ We__ Th__ Fr__ Sa__ Su__

Dinner

Food/ Beverage	Serving Size	Sodium	Calories	Protein	Carbs	Fat
Totals						

Snack

Serving size _____   _____ Protein

Sodium _____   _____ Carbs

Calories _____   _____ Fat

Notes

Misc. Info

Date: _____

Mo__ Tu__ We__ Th__ Fr__ Sa__ Su__

Breakfast

Food/ Beverage	Serving Size	Sodium	Calories	Protein	Carbs	Fat
Totals						

Snack

Serving size _____   _____ Protein

Sodium _____   _____ Carbs

Calories _____   _____ Fat

Notes

Misc. Info

Date: _____

Mo__ Tu__ We__ Th__ Fr__ Sa__ Su__

Lunch

Food/ Beverage	Serving Size	Sodium	Calories	Protein	Carbs	Fat
Totals						

Snack

Serving size _____   _____ Protein

Sodium _____   _____ Carbs

Calories _____   _____ Fat

Notes

Misc. Info

Date: _____

Mo__ Tu__ We__ Th__ Fr__ Sa__ Su__

Dinner

Food/ Beverage	Serving Size	Sodium	Calories	Protein	Carbs	Fat
Totals						

Snack

Serving size _____

Sodium _____

Calories _____

_____ Protein

_____ Carbs

_____ Fat

Notes

Misc. Info

Date: _____

Mo__ Tu__ We__ Th__ Fr__ Sa__ Su__

Breakfast

Food/ Beverage	Serving Size	Sodium	Calories	Protein	Carbs	Fat
Totals						

Snack

Serving size _____   _____ Protein

Sodium _____   _____ Carbs

Calories _____   _____ Fat

Notes

Misc. Info

Date: _____, ___

Mo__ Tu__ We__ Th__ Fr__ Sa__ Su__

Lunch

Food/ Beverage	Serving Size	Sodium	Calories	Protein	Carbs	Fat
Totals						

Snack

Serving size _____   _____ Protein

Sodium _____   _____ Carbs

Calories _____   _____ Fat

Notes

Misc. Info

Date: _____

Mo__ Tu__ We__ Th__ Fr__ Sa__ Su__

Dinner

Food/ Beverage	Serving Size	Sodium	Calories	Protein	Carbs	Fat
Totals						

Snack

Serving size _____   _____ Protein

Sodium   _____   _____ Carbs

Calories   _____   _____ Fat

Notes

Misc. Info

Date: _____

Mo__ Tu__ We__ Th__ Fr__ Sa__ Su__

Breakfast

Food/ Beverage	Serving Size	Sodium	Calories	Protein	Carbs	Fat
Totals						

Snack

Serving size _____   _____ Protein

Sodium   _____   _____ Carbs

Calories   _____   _____ Fat

Notes

Misc. Info

Date: _____

Mo__ Tu__ We__ Th__ Fr__ Sa__ Su__

Breakfast

Food/ Beverage	Serving Size	Sodium	Calories	Protein	Carbs	Fat
Totals						

Snack

Serving size _____   _____ Protein

Sodium   _____   _____ Carbs

Calories   _____   _____ Fat

Notes

Misc. Info

Date: _____

Mo__ Tu__ We__ Th__ Fr__ Sa__ Su__

Lunch

Food/ Beverage	Serving Size	Sodium	Calories	Protein	Carbs	Fat
Totals						

Snack

Serving size _____   _____ Protein

Sodium   _____   _____ Carbs

Calories   _____   _____ Fat

Notes

Misc. Info

Date: _____

Mo__ Tu__ We__ Th__ Fr__ Sa__ Su__

Dinner

Food/ Beverage	Serving Size	Sodium	Calories	Protein	Carbs	Fat
Totals						

Snack

Serving size _____   _____ Protein

Sodium   _____   _____ Carbs

Calories   _____   _____ Fat

Notes

Misc. Info

Date: _____

Mo__ Tu__ We__ Th__ Fr__ Sa__ Su__

Breakfast

Food/ Beverage	Serving Size	Sodium	Calories	Protein	Carbs	Fat
Totals						

Snack

Serving size _____   _____ Protein

Sodium   _____   _____ Carbs

Calories   _____   _____ Fat

Notes

Misc. Info

Date: _____

Mo__ Tu__ We__ Th__ Fr__ Sa__ Su__

Lunch

Food/ Beverage	Serving Size	Sodium	Calories	Protein	Carbs	Fat
Totals						

Snack

Serving size _____   _____ Protein

Sodium   _____   _____ Carbs

Calories   _____   _____ Fat

Notes

Misc. Info

Date: _____

Mo__ Tu__ We__ Th__ Fr__ Sa__ Su__

Dinner

Food/ Beverage	Serving Size	Sodium	Calories	Protein	Carbs	Fat
Totals						

Snack

Serving size _____   _____ Protein

Sodium   _____   _____ Carbs

Calories   _____   _____ Fat

Notes

Misc. Info

Date: _____

Mo__ Tu__ We__ Th__ Fr__ Sa__ Su__

Breakfast

Food/ Beverage	Serving Size	Sodium	Calories	Protein	Carbs	Fat
Totals						

Snack

Serving size _____   _____ Protein

Sodium   _____   _____ Carbs

Calories   _____   _____ Fat

Notes

Misc. Info

Date: _____

Mo__ Tu__ We__ Th__ Fr__ Sa__ Su__

Lunch

Food/ Beverage	Serving Size	Sodium	Calories	Protein	Carbs	Fat
Totals						

Snack

Serving size _____   _____ Protein

Sodium   _____   _____ Carbs

Calories   _____   _____ Fat

Notes

Misc. Info

Date: _____

Mo__ Tu__ We__ Th__ Fr__ Sa__ Su__

Dinner

Food/ Beverage	Serving Size	Sodium	Calories	Protein	Carbs	Fat
Totals						

Snack

Serving size _____   _____ Protein

Sodium   _____   _____ Carbs

Calories   _____   _____ Fat

Notes

Misc. Info

Date: _____

Mo__ Tu__ We__ Th__ Fr__ Sa__ Su__

Breakfast

Food/ Beverage	Serving Size	Sodium	Calories	Protein	Carbs	Fat
Totals						

Snack

Serving size _____   _____ Protein

Sodium _____   _____ Carbs

Calories _____   _____ Fat

Notes

Misc. Info

Date: _____

Mo__ Tu__ We__ Th__ Fr__ Sa__ Su__

Lunch

Food/ Beverage	Serving Size	Sodium	Calories	Protein	Carbs	Fat
Totals						

Snack

Serving size _____   _____ Protein

Sodium _____   _____ Carbs

Calories _____   _____ Fat

Notes

Misc. Info

Date: _____

Mo__ Tu__ We__ Th__ Fr__ Sa__ Su__

Dinner

Food/ Beverage	Serving Size	Sodium	Calories	Protein	Carbs	Fat
Totals						

Snack

Serving size _____   _____ Protein

Sodium   _____   _____ Carbs

Calories   _____   _____ Fat

Notes

Misc. Info

Date: _____

Mo__ Tu__ We__ Th__ Fr__ Sa__ Su__

Breakfast

Food/ Beverage	Serving Size	Sodium	Calories	Protein	Carbs	Fat
Totals						

Snack

Serving size _____   _____ Protein
Sodium   _____   _____ Carbs
Calories   _____   _____ Fat

Notes

Misc. Info

Date: _____

Mo__ Tu__ We__ Th__ Fr__ Sa__ Su__

Lunch

Food/ Beverage	Serving Size	Sodium	Calories	Protein	Carbs	Fat
Totals						

Snack

Serving size _____   _____ Protein

Sodium _____   _____ Carbs

Calories _____   _____ Fat

Notes

Misc. Info

Date: _____

Mo__ Tu__ We__ Th__ Fr__ Sa__ Su__

Dinner

Food/ Beverage	Serving Size	Sodium	Calories	Protein	Carbs	Fat
Totals						

Snack

Serving size _____   _____ Protein

Sodium _____   _____ Carbs

Calories _____   _____ Fat

Notes

Misc. Info

Date: _____

Mo__ Tu__ We__ Th__ Fr__ Sa__ Su__

Breakfast

Food/ Beverage	Serving Size	Sodium	Calories	Protein	Carbs	Fat
Totals						

Snack

Serving size _____   _____ Protein

Sodium _____   _____ Carbs

Calories _____   _____ Fat

Notes

Misc. Info

Date: _____

Mo__ Tu__ We__ Th__ Fr__ Sa__ Su__

Lunch

Food/ Beverage	Serving Size	Sodium	Calories	Protein	Carbs	Fat
Totals						

Snack

Serving size _____   _____ Protein

Sodium   _____   _____ Carbs

Calories   _____   _____ Fat

Notes

Misc. Info

Date: _____

Mo__ Tu__ We__ Th__ Fr__ Sa__ Su__

Dinner

Food/ Beverage	Serving Size	Sodium	Calories	Protein	Carbs	Fat
Totals						

Snack

Serving size _____   _____ Protein

Sodium   _____   _____ Carbs

Calories   _____   _____ Fat

Notes

Misc. Info

Date: _____

Mo__ Tu__ We__ Th__ Fr__ Sa__ Su__

Breakfast

Food/ Beverage	Serving Size	Sodium	Calories	Protein	Carbs	Fat
Totals						

Snack

Serving size _____   _____ Protein

Sodium _____   _____ Carbs

Calories _____   _____ Fat

Notes

Misc. Info

Date: _____

Mo__ Tu__ We__ Th__ Fr__ Sa__ Su__

Lunch

Food/ Beverage	Serving Size	Sodium	Calories	Protein	Carbs	Fat
Totals						

Snack

Serving size _____   _____ Protein

Sodium   _____   _____ Carbs

Calories   _____   _____ Fat

Notes

Misc. Info

Date: _____

Mo__ Tu__ We__ Th__ Fr__ Sa__ Su__

Dinner

Food/ Beverage	Serving Size	Sodium	Calories	Protein	Carbs	Fat
Totals						

Snack

Serving size _____   _____ Protein

Sodium   _____   _____ Carbs

Calories   _____   _____ Fat

Notes

Misc. Info

Date: _____

Mo__ Tu__ We__ Th__ Fr__ Sa__ Su__

Breakfast

Food/ Beverage	Serving Size	Sodium	Calories	Protein	Carbs	Fat
Totals						

Snack

Serving size _____   _____ Protein

Sodium   _____   _____ Carbs

Calories   _____   _____ Fat

Notes

Misc. Info

Date: _____

Mo__ Tu__ We__ Th__ Fr__ Sa__ Su__

Lunch

Food/ Beverage	Serving Size	Sodium	Calories	Protein	Carbs	Fat
Totals						

Snack

Serving size _____   _____ Protein

Sodium   _____   _____ Carbs

Calories   _____   _____ Fat

Notes

Misc. Info

Date: _____

Mo__ Tu__ We__ Th__ Fr__ Sa__ Su__

Dinner

Food/ Beverage	Serving Size	Sodium	Calories	Protein	Carbs	Fat
Totals						

Snack

Serving size _____   _____ Protein

Sodium _____   _____ Carbs

Calories _____   _____ Fat

Notes

Misc. Info

Date: _____

Mo__ Tu__ We__ Th__ Fr__ Sa__ Su__

Breakfast

Food/ Beverage	Serving Size	Sodium	Calories	Protein	Carbs	Fat
Totals						

Snack

Serving size _____   _____ Protein

Sodium _____   _____ Carbs

Calories _____   _____ Fat

Notes

Misc. Info

Date: _____

Mo__ Tu__ We__ Th__ Fr__ Sa__ Su__

Lunch

Food/ Beverage	Serving Size	Sodium	Calories	Protein	Carbs	Fat
Totals						

Snack

Serving size _____   _____ Protein

Sodium   _____   _____ Carbs

Calories   _____   _____ Fat

Notes

Misc. Info

Date: _____

Mo__ Tu__ We__ Th__ Fr__ Sa__ Su__

Dinner

Food/ Beverage	Serving Size	Sodium	Calories	Protein	Carbs	Fat
Totals						

Snack

Serving size _____   _____ Protein

Sodium _____   _____ Carbs

Calories _____   _____ Fat

Notes

Misc. Info

Date: _____

Mo__ Tu__ We__ Th__ Fr__ Sa__ Su__

Breakfast

Food/ Beverage	Serving Size	Sodium	Calories	Protein	Carbs	Fat
Totals						

Snack

Serving size _____   _____ Protein

Sodium   _____   _____ Carbs

Calories   _____   _____ Fat

Notes

Misc. Info

Date: _____

Mo__ Tu__ We__ Th__ Fr__ Sa__ Su__

Lunch

Food/ Beverage	Serving Size	Sodium	Calories	Protein	Carbs	Fat
Totals						

Snack

Serving size _____   _____ Protein

Sodium   _____   _____ Carbs

Calories   _____   _____ Fat

Notes

Misc. Info

Date: _____

Mo__ Tu__ We__ Th__ Fr__ Sa__ Su__

Dinner

Food/ Beverage	Serving Size	Sodium	Calories	Protein	Carbs	Fat
Totals						

Snack

Serving size _____   _____ Protein

Sodium   _____   _____ Carbs

Calories   _____   _____ Fat

Notes

Misc. Info

Date: _____

Mo__ Tu__ We__ Th__ Fr__ Sa__ Su__

Breakfast

Food/ Beverage	Serving Size	Sodium	Calories	Protein	Carbs	Fat
Totals						

Snack

Serving size _____   _____ Protein

Sodium   _____   _____ Carbs

Calories   _____   _____ Fat

Notes

Misc. Info

Date: _____

Mo__ Tu__ We__ Th__ Fr__ Sa__ Su__

Lunch

Food/ Beverage	Serving Size	Sodium	Calories	Protein	Carbs	Fat
Totals						

Snack

Serving size _____   _____ Protein

Sodium _____   _____ Carbs

Calories _____   _____ Fat

Notes

Misc. Info

Date: _____

Mo__ Tu__ We__ Th__ Fr__ Sa__ Su__

Dinner

Food/ Beverage	Serving Size	Sodium	Calories	Protein	Carbs	Fat
Totals						

Snack

Serving size _____   _____ Protein

Sodium   _____   _____ Carbs

Calories   _____   _____ Fat

Notes

Misc. Info

Date: _____

Mo__ Tu__ We__ Th__ Fr__ Sa__ Su__

Breakfast

Food/ Beverage	Serving Size	Sodium	Calories	Protein	Carbs	Fat
Totals						

Snack

Serving size _____   _____ Protein

Sodium   _____   _____ Carbs

Calories   _____   _____ Fat

Notes

Misc. Info

Date: _____

Mo__ Tu__ We__ Th__ Fr__ Sa__ Su__

Lunch

Food/ Beverage	Serving Size	Sodium	Calories	Protein	Carbs	Fat
Totals						

Snack

Serving size _____   _____ Protein

Sodium   _____   _____ Carbs

Calories   _____   _____ Fat

Notes

Misc. Info

Date: _____

Mo__ Tu__ We__ Th__ Fr__ Sa__ Su__

Dinner

Food/ Beverage	Serving Size	Sodium	Calories	Protein	Carbs	Fat
Totals						

Snack

Serving size _____   _____ Protein

Sodium   _____   _____ Carbs

Calories   _____   _____ Fat

Notes

Misc. Info

Date: _____

Mo__ Tu__ We__ Th__ Fr__ Sa__ Su__

Breakfast

Food/ Beverage	Serving Size	Sodium	Calories	Protein	Carbs	Fat
Totals						

Snack

Serving size _____   _____ Protein

Sodium   _____   _____ Carbs

Calories   _____   _____ Fat

Notes

Misc. Info

Date: _____

Mo__ Tu__ We__ Th__ Fr__ Sa__ Su__

Breakfast

Food/ Beverage	Serving Size	Sodium	Calories	Protein	Carbs	Fat
Totals						

Snack

Serving size _____   _____ Protein

Sodium   _____   _____ Carbs

Calories   _____   _____ Fat

Notes

Misc. Info

Date: _____

Mo__ Tu__ We__ Th__ Fr__ Sa__ Su__

Lunch

Food/ Beverage	Serving Size	Sodium	Calories	Protein	Carbs	Fat
Totals						

Snack

Serving size _____   _____ Protein

Sodium   _____   _____ Carbs

Calories   _____   _____ Fat

Notes

Misc. Info

Date: _____

Mo__ Tu__ We__ Th__ Fr__ Sa__ Su__

Dinner

Food/ Beverage	Serving Size	Sodium	Calories	Protein	Carbs	Fat
Totals						

Snack

Serving size _____   _____ Protein

Sodium   _____   _____ Carbs

Calories   _____   _____ Fat

Notes

Misc. Info

Date: _____

Mo__ Tu__ We__ Th__ Fr__ Sa__ Su__

Breakfast

Food/ Beverage	Serving Size	Sodium	Calories	Protein	Carbs	Fat
Totals						

Snack

Serving size _____   _____ Protein

Sodium _____   _____ Carbs

Calories _____   _____ Fat

Notes

Misc. Info

Date: _____

Mo__ Tu__ We__ Th__ Fr__ Sa__ Su__

Lunch

Food/ Beverage	Serving Size	Sodium	Calories	Protein	Carbs	Fat
Totals						

Snack

Serving size _____   _____ Protein

Sodium   _____   _____ Carbs

Calories   _____   _____ Fat

Notes

Misc. Info

Date: _____

Mo__ Tu__ We__ Th__ Fr__ Sa__ Su__

Dinner

Food/ Beverage	Serving Size	Sodium	Calories	Protein	Carbs	Fat
Totals						

Snack

Serving size _____   _____ Protein

Sodium   _____   _____ Carbs

Calories   _____   _____ Fat

Notes

Misc. Info

Date: _____

Mo__ Tu__ We__ Th__ Fr__ Sa__ Su__

Breakfast

Food/ Beverage	Serving Size	Sodium	Calories	Protein	Carbs	Fat
Totals						

Snack

Serving size _____   _____ Protein

Sodium   _____   _____ Carbs

Calories   _____   _____ Fat

Notes

Misc. Info

Date: _____

Mo__ Tu__ We__ Th__ Fr__ Sa__ Su__

Lunch

Food/ Beverage	Serving Size	Sodium	Calories	Protein	Carbs	Fat
Totals						

Snack

Serving size _____   _____ Protein

Sodium _____   _____ Carbs

Calories _____   _____ Fat

Notes

Misc. Info

Date: _____

Mo__ Tu__ We__ Th__ Fr__ Sa__ Su__

Dinner

Food/ Beverage	Serving Size	Sodium	Calories	Protein	Carbs	Fat
Totals						

Snack

Serving size _____   _____ Protein

Sodium _____   _____ Carbs

Calories _____   _____ Fat

Notes

Misc. Info

Date: _____

Mo__ Tu__ We__ Th__ Fr__ Sa__ Su__

Breakfast

Food/ Beverage	Serving Size	Sodium	Calories	Protein	Carbs	Fat
Totals						

Snack

Serving size _____   _____ Protein

Sodium   _____   _____ Carbs

Calories   _____   _____ Fat

Notes

Misc. Info

Date: _____

Mo__ Tu__ We__ Th__ Fr__ Sa__ Su__

Lunch

Food/ Beverage	Serving Size	Sodium	Calories	Protein	Carbs	Fat
Totals						

Snack

Serving size _____   _____ Protein

Sodium _____   _____ Carbs

Calories _____   _____ Fat

Notes

Misc. Info

Date: _____

Mo__ Tu__ We__ Th__ Fr__ Sa__ Su__

Dinner

Food/ Beverage	Serving Size	Sodium	Calories	Protein	Carbs	Fat
Totals						

Snack

Serving size _____   _____ Protein

Sodium   _____   _____ Carbs

Calories _____   _____ Fat

Notes

Misc. Info

Date: _____

Mo__ Tu__ We__ Th__ Fr__ Sa__ Su__

Breakfast

Food/ Beverage	Serving Size	Sodium	Calories	Protein	Carbs	Fat
Totals						

Snack

Serving size _____   _____ Protein

Sodium   _____   _____ Carbs

Calories   _____   _____ Fat

Notes

Misc. Info

Date: _____

Mo__ Tu__ We__ Th__ Fr__ Sa__ Su__

Lunch

Food/ Beverage	Serving Size	Sodium	Calories	Protein	Carbs	Fat
Totals						

Snack

Serving size _____   _____ Protein

Sodium _____   _____ Carbs

Calories _____   _____ Fat

Notes

Misc. Info

Date: _____

Mo__ Tu__ We__ Th__ Fr__ Sa__ Su__

Dinner

Food/ Beverage	Serving Size	Sodium	Calories	Protein	Carbs	Fat
Totals						

Snack

Serving size _____

Sodium _____

Calories _____

_____ Protein

_____ Carbs

_____ Fat

Notes

Misc. Info

Date: _____

Mo__ Tu__ We__ Th__ Fr__ Sa__ Su__

Breakfast

Food/Beverage	Serving Size	Sodium	Calories	Protein	Carbs	Fat
Totals						

Snack

Serving size _____   _____ Protein

Sodium   _____   _____ Carbs

Calories   _____   _____ Fat

Notes

Misc. Info

Date: _____

Mo__ Tu__ We__ Th__ Fr__ Sa__ Su__

Lunch

Food/Beverage	Serving Size	Sodium	Calories	Protein	Carbs	Fat
Totals						

Snack

Serving size _____   _____ Protein

Sodium _____   _____ Carbs

Calories _____   _____ Fat

Notes

Misc. Info

Date: _____

Mo__ Tu__ We__ Th__ Fr__ Sa__ Su__

Dinner

Food/ Beverage	Serving Size	Sodium	Calories	Protein	Carbs	Fat
Totals						

Snack

Serving size _____   _____ Protein

Sodium   _____   _____ Carbs

Calories   _____   _____ Fat

Notes

Misc. Info

Notes

Introduction

1. Heister, Chantel. The "Top 10 Reasons for a Low Sodium Diet." *SYNERGY HomeCare,* 17 June 2011. https://www.synergyhomecare.com/blog/posts/2011/6/17/the-top-10-reasons-for-a-low-sodium-diet/#.W8CTfGNN5PY. Accessed 12 October 2018.

2. "Sodium and Food Sources." National Center for Chronic Disease Prevention and Health Promotion, Division for Heart Disease and Stroke Prevention, 28 March 2017. https://www.cdc.gov/salt/food.htm. Accessed 12 October 2018.

3. "Sodium sources: Where does all that sodium come from?" American Heart Association, 23 May 2018. https://www.heart.org/en/healthy-living/healthy-eating/eat-smart/sodium/sodium-sources. Accessed 15 October 2018.

Made in the USA
Middletown, DE
31 May 2020